I AM EMPOWER

The Path from Trauma to Truth

Mahsa Khodabakhsh, D.C., B.S., B.M.Sc., C.Hyp

I Am Empower
The Path from Trauma to Truth

Published by Reflek Publishing

Disclaimer: The author makes no guarantees concerning the level of success you may experience by following the advice and strategies contained in this book, and you accept the risk that results will differ for each individual. The purpose of this book is to educate, entertain, and inspire.

For more information: info@drmahsa.com

ISBN: 978-1-968164-40-9 (paperback)
ISBN: 978-1-968164-41-6 (ebook)

Love heals. And you are love.

—Dr. Mahsa

Dedication

This book is dedicated to anyone
who has ever felt disempowered.

All the power you will ever need
is already within you.

Remember: love heals, and you are Love.

Here's a free gift before you begin!

You've picked up this book.
Now it's time to find your truth.

Here's a free gift to help you begin your journey:

A companion guide and a downloadable
hypno-breathwork session,
made just for you!

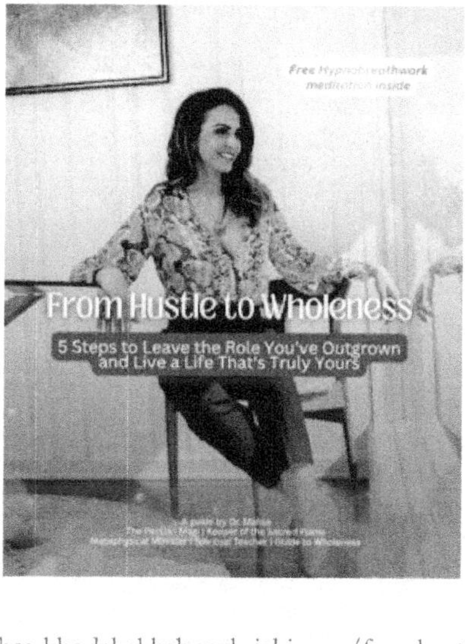

https://mahsa-khodabakhsh.mykajabi.com/fromhustletowholeness

Table of contents

Introduction

This Book Is for You

Maybe you picked up this book and weren't even sure why. Something just pulled you toward it—a quiet tug you couldn't explain. That pull was not random. That pull was your soul, recognizing something it has been waiting to find.

This book is for you. Whoever you are. Whatever you've survived. However long you've been carrying what was never yours to carry.

You already know. You felt it the moment you read the first line.

This book is for the one who was told they were too much, and for the one who was told they weren't enough. For the child who was told they couldn't dance, sing, show their face—who couldn't be *free*. For anyone who has been silenced, shamed, or shrunk down to fit into spaces that were never meant to contain them.

For anyone who has been physically abused and told they deserved it. Who believed, even for a moment, that the violence was their fault. For every soul across the world who carries the same invisible chains—different countries, different cultures, same cage.

This book is for the wild hearts who love passionately, who feel deeply, and who are told their intensity is a flaw instead of their greatest gift. For the dancers who were told they can't move their bodies. The singers who were told to be quiet. The artists who were told to be practical. The dreamers who were told to wake up.

For the lovers who couldn't show their love. Who hid the most beautiful thing about being human—the capacity to connect, to feel, to touch, to adore. And for those who feel called to empower others.

This book is for you.

How I Found My Way

I first noticed Michael when I was a freshman in high school and he was a senior.

A month before our mutual birthdays—my twentieth and his twenty-third—he died in a tragic accident.

In a love letter he left behind, he wrote five words that became the foundation of everything I now believe about healing, about love, about what it means to be human:

"I am love for you."

I carried those words through grief, through trauma, through years of darkness I didn't think I would survive. And slowly, painfully, beautifully—they changed everything.

Love is not something you find. It is something you *are*. That truth became my compass. It led me out of grief. It led me into healing, into a life of service. And it is the truth at the heart of this book.

Why I Wrote This Book

I wrote this book for the little girl in me and for people all across the world who have had their basic human rights stripped from them.

I wrote it for the women of Iran—the ones who came before me and the ones who are still there now, still fighting, still resisting, still paying with their lives for the simple audacity of wanting to be free. The young women in the streets. The mothers. The students. The ones who removed their hijabs in public and were arrested. The ones who chanted and were shot. The ones whose names we may never know but whose courage lives in all of us who got out of Iran but never forgot what we went through and those we had to leave behind—grandparents, parents, sisters, brothers, cousins, and friends whom we loved dearly.

This book is my living room dance. My Michael Jackson video from the black market. My act of defiance and devotion—to every soul that was told it could not move, could not speak, could not shine.

I know that soul. I was her.

I was the one who danced in secret behind closed doors, terrified of being seen, of bringing harm to her family, of being punished for the simple natural act of moving her body to music. The one who carried that fear in her cells long after she left Iran. Long after she came to America. Long after she was supposedly "free."

Even in freedom, I found new cages. Cages of shame. Cages of unworthiness. Cages of other people's judgments and expectations. Cages I built myself because I didn't yet know my own power.

I spent years feeling not enough. Questioning my worth. Dimming my light to make others comfortable, to be accepted. Giving my power away and allowing people in my life who didn't deserve me.

And then, painfully and beautifully—I woke up. Not in a dramatic revelation, but in an ordinary afternoon when the light was falling a certain way, I remembered. Something ancient. Something that had been true about me since before I had language for it.

I am divine. I am powerful. I am love, walking around in a human body, temporarily confused about what I am. And if you are reading this, so are you.

This remembering didn't happen overnight. It happened through years of inner work—through healing my body, through meditation and spiritual practice, through facing my shadows and integrating my pain, through studying the traditions of ancient wisdom and the metaphysical laws that govern our universe.

Love has been my message for as long as I can remember. Love is medicine. Love heals. Love is who we are at our very core. And empowerment is what happens when you finally remember that you are love. When you know you are love, you stop giving your power away. You stop accepting treatment you don't deserve. You stop hiding, shrinking, and dimming your light.

First, these were words I spoke to myself in the mirror, trying to believe them. Then, when I opened my chiropractic clinic, I named it "Empowered"—because I wanted to help my patients remember the power already within them. But really it was I who wanted to be empowered. Empowerment became my life's work. But love has always been the root. And now, both have become this book.

If any part of my story lives in you . . . if you have ever felt too much, or not enough, or simply forgotten who you truly are . . . this book is for you. We all have our cages. We all have our battles. And we all have within us the same divine spark that is waiting—patiently, lovingly, with infinite faith in you—to be remembered.

This book is your invitation home.

What I Am EMPOWER Means

The title of this book is not a statement about being empowered by something outside yourself.

I AM are the two most powerful words in any language. They are the words the Divine used to name itself. They are the words that, when followed by anything, create your reality. EMPOWER is not a gift given to you. It is a truth you remember. I AM EMPOWER means the power has always been within you. The wisdom has always been within you. The divine has always been within you. This book simply helps you remember what you already know.

What You Will Discover

This book is organized around the acronym EMPOWER—seven sacred tools for transformation:

E—Energy: You are not just flesh and bone. You are a vibrational being, and your thoughts, words, and emotions are constantly creating your reality.

M—Meditation: The practice of getting quiet enough to hear your soul and connect with the infinite intelligence that has always lived within you.

P—Presence: The greatest gift you can give, to yourself and to others, is your full, undivided attention.

O—Oneness: We are not separate beings bumping into each other on a random planet. We are one consciousness expressing itself through infinite forms.

W—Wisdom: The innate knowing that lives in your bones, your gut, your heart, older and truer than anything you were ever taught.

E—Evolution: Your soul came here to grow. Your struggles were not punishments. They were preparation.

R—Reveal: The final act of healing is letting the world see who you truly are. No more hiding. No more shrinking. No more performing.

How to Read This Book

You can read this book from beginning to end, or you can open it to wherever you are called. Each chapter stands on its own and also builds on what came before.

At the end of each chapter, you will find exercises. Please do them. The transformation in this book is not intellectual; it is experiential. You cannot think your way into healing. You must feel your way there.

Bring a journal. Bring an open heart. Bring the willingness to be honest with yourself. That is all you need. Let's begin.

I AM here.
I AM ready.
I AM coming home.

E: Energy

If you want to find the secrets of the universe, think in terms of energy, frequency and vibration.

—Nikola Tesla

Some of what I share in this chapter you may have heard before. These are universal laws and principles—spoken about and taught by mystics, philosophers, scientists, and New Thought teachers across centuries and cultures. There is a reason they keep being rediscovered: because they are true. Universal laws don't belong to any one tradition or teacher. They belong to all of us.

I am not here to hand you a textbook. I am here to share what these laws have looked and felt like lived from the inside—in the moments that broke me open, held me back, brought me to my knees, and ultimately set me free. Because learning about the universe is one thing. Truly experiencing it is something else entirely. It is calming. It is miraculous. It awakens the soul in a way that no amount of reading ever quite can.

Over the years I have come to understand (through living, not just studying) that my energy and my state of being completely shifts my experience of everything. The same circumstances can feel entirely different, depending on where I am inside myself. And I have also learned that some of the most seemingly unfair things that happened to me were, in fact, gifts. Invitations. Teachings dressed up as disasters.

Once I began to let go of fear—to truly let go, not just to intellectually understand that I should—everything started to feel different.

I want to be honest with you, though: I am still a human being who makes mistakes. The difference now is that when something feels off, I get curious instead of just suffering through it. I ask myself: Why did this show up? What was I thinking, speaking, feeling in the days before this? Was I balanced and at peace—or was I running on empty, letting fear or resentment quietly run the show?

Because here is what I have noticed, in myself and in the thousands of patients I have sat with over the years: When we are exhausted and haven't allowed ourselves to rest and truly recuperate, our energy drops. And low energy doesn't just affect us; it also radiates outward. It touches everyone around us.

You have felt this. Think about the last time you were truly depleted and had to push through anyway. How heavy did everything feel? Now think about a time when you were well rested, doing something that lit you up, surrounded by people who felt good to be near. Same life. Completely different energy.

Sadly, we have built a world that keeps most people in the first state far more often than the second. We are burned out. Overwhelmed. Constantly bombarded with fear—in the news, on our screens, in the conversations swirling around us. And fear pulls us away from love. From our true nature. It lowers our frequency, clouds our perception, and quietly convinces us that we are powerless.

What we see, as a result, is a world full of people who are exhausted, reactive, judgmental, and afraid—not because that is who they are but because they have forgotten what they are made of.

One of my favorite books is Marianne Williamson's *A Return to Love*—a beautiful, luminous guide back to what matters most. Her central teaching, drawn from *A Course in Miracles*, is elegantly simple. There are only two emotions: love and fear. And fear is a call for love.[1] This chapter is about the choice to be *love*, and about the energy that flows from it.

---

1. Marianne Williamson . *A Return to Love: Reflections on the Principles of A Course in Miracles*. (HarperCollins, 1992)

You Are Made of Energy

Try this right now: Rub your hands together fast. Notice the heat building up. Do this for about twenty to thirty seconds, then gently move your hands away from each other.

Do you notice a pull or a density? A heat or a vibration between your palms? This is your energy. The natural vibration is created by your body's frequency. And this energy is powerful. It is healing.

Reiki[2] is an example of this, but it doesn't need to be Reiki. We can command and move energy with intention and thought, especially when combining the brain-and-heart connection. This is the foundation of all healing work: the energy already flowing through you. All life is energy.

The late hypnotherapist Dolores Cannon spent over forty years conducting thousands of deep-hypnosis sessions around the world. What she found consistently—across cultures, languages, and lifetimes—was this: Every subject, when brought to the deepest level of their own consciousness, reported the same thing. We are all made of the same energy. We come from the same Source. The separation we feel between ourselves and others, between ourselves and the Divine, is the illusion. What is real is the energy that connects everything.[3] I found her work

2. Japanese energy healing system developed by Mikao Usui in the early twentieth century.

3. Dolores Cannon, *The Convoluted Universe* (Ozark Mountain Publishing, 2001-2013).

remarkable because it confirmed what ancient wisdom has always known—and what your body already feels when you rub your hands together and sense that invisible pull.

The Hermetic Principle of Mentalism

The ancient Hermetic teachings,[4] which predates modern science by thousands of years, begins with this principle: The All is Mind. The Universe is Mental.

The fundamental nature of reality is consciousness, not matter. Mind is primary. Everything else is secondary. Science finally caught up to what mystics always knew. At the subatomic level, particles do not exist in fixed states until they are *observed.* Consciousness shapes matter. Your attention is not passive; it is a creative force. The act of simply witnessing something changes it. You are not a passive observer of your life. You are an active creator of it.

Every thought you think is energy. Every word you speak is energy. Every emotion you feel is energy. And all of it is broadcasting outward, attracting circumstances, people, and experiences that match its frequency. This is the mechanism of creation.

---

4. The Seven Hermetic Principles originate from the ancient Egyptian-Greek tradition attributed to Hermes Trismegistus, preserved in *The Kybalion* and related texts.

Your Body Is Energy

Your body is not a machine. It is a living broadcast, every organ humming its own note, every cell constantly conversing with the field around it. You extend beyond your skin. You always have.

You have walked into a room and felt the energy shift. You have met someone and felt an immediate sense of ease—or an immediate sense of warning. You have held a grieving friend and felt their sorrow move through you. You have been in the presence of someone joyful and felt yourself lighten. This is not imagination. This is something older than language, the ability to read what cannot be seen, to know what cannot be explained. The question is whether you trust what you feel.

How Trauma Lives in the Body

When you experience trauma, it doesn't just affect your mind. It lives in your body.

The nervous system responds to threat by mobilizing energy: fight, flight, or freeze. When the threat passes and the energy is not discharged, it gets stored. In the muscles. In the fascia. In the organs. In the cellular memory. This is why you can know intellectually that you are safe and still feel terrified. This is why you can understand that your past is over and still react as though it is happening now. The body holds what the mind has not yet processed.

This is also why healing must be somatic—in the body—not just cognitive. Movement, breath, touch, sound . . . these are not luxuries. They are medicine.

Louise Hay taught this for decades: Illness does not begin in the body. It begins in the energy field. The physical symptom is the last stop on a long journey that started in unprocessed emotion, unresolved fear, and unexpressed truth. The body is always trying to communicate. Disease is information.[5]

This is exactly what I have witnessed in sixteen years of clinical practice. The back gives out under the weight of a life someone has been carrying alone. The gut rebels when boundaries keep being swallowed. The chest tightens around a grief that was never given permission to exist. The body does not lie. It has simply been waiting for someone to ask the right questions.

When My Body Carried Everything

I was five months pregnant with my son when I slipped out of the bathtub and fell hard onto the bathroom tile. I broke my sacrum and coccyx—my back. I was a chiropractor with a broken back and a baby on the way. The irony was not lost on me. And I was terrified.

5. Louise L. Hay, *You Can Heal Your Life* (Hay House, 1984).

But the fall was only one layer of what I was carrying. At the same time, I was being harassed by an unstable patient. The fear this created in me was unlike anything I had experienced before. It lived in my chest, in my nervous system, in every cell of my body. And on top of that, there was the financial stress of not being able to work, the physical pain of my injury, and the constant, looping question that I could not silence:

Is my baby going to be okay?

I understood the nervous system. I understood stress physiology. I understood that what a mother feels, her body transmits—and that what her body transmits, her baby receives. I knew all of this. And I could not stop feeling afraid.

So I did everything I knew how to do. I meditated. I visualized. I practiced self-hypnosis. I focused my attention on one image: a healthy baby boy, born whole and breathing. I surrendered myself to the Creator, to the Universe, to God—whatever name you give to that forçe greater than ourselves.

When he was born, he wasn't breathing.

The silence in that delivery room was the longest silence of my life.

And then, finally, a small cry. He was alive.

In the months that followed, he developed eczema and severe allergies. He was sensitive in ways I hadn't anticipated.

And I carried tremendous guilt. I blamed myself: the stress I was under, the fall, the fear I couldn't stop feeling while pregnant. Somehow, my body had transmitted all of that into his tiny, perfect body.

About two years later, that same unstable patient reappeared in my life. Bringing the same imagined accusations, and the same energy of threat. And something in me was triggered all over again. Every fear I had held during that pregnancy came flooding back.

I believe that what we speak and vocalize, we bring into existence. So I don't like to dwell on these circumstances. But I share this because it taught me something I needed to understand: The energy of fear—when it is not processed, when it is suppressed and carried in the body—continues to move. It doesn't disappear. It looks for somewhere to go.

Over time, through consistent work (calming my nervous system, addressing my son's sensitivities with care, practicing energy work, and releasing the guilt and the fear I had been holding for him having suffered), his allergies improved. His eczema healed. He became more settled. Not overnight. Not magically. But progressively.

The fear I carried during that pregnancy was real. The guilt that followed was real. But so was the love. And it was the love—turned inward, practiced daily, offered to myself as medicine—that ultimately moved what fear had frozen.

The body always knows how to come home to itself when given the chance.

And the unstable patient, I sent her love too.

The Principle of Vibration

Everything vibrates. Nothing rests. This is the Hermetic Principle of Vibration, and it has profound implications for how you live.

Your emotional states are frequencies. Fear vibrates low. Love vibrates high. Shame, guilt, and grief sit at the bottom of the scale. Joy, gratitude, and love sit at the top. Wherever you vibrate most consistently, that is what you attract into your life. This is not about toxic positivity or pretending you don't feel what you feel. It is about understanding that your emotional state is your point of attraction and that you have more influence over it than you have been taught. When you shift your vibration, you shift your reality.

The Principle of Polarity

Everything has an opposite. Hot and cold are the same thing—temperature—at different degrees. Love and fear are opposites on the same spectrum. Light and shadow cannot exist without each other.

This principle liberates you from the war against yourself. You do not need to eliminate your darkness. You need to understand it. Your fear is not your enemy; it is energy that has not yet been transformed. Your anger is a signal pointing to something that needs your attention. Your grief is love with nowhere to go.

When you stop fighting your so-called negative emotions and start listening to them, they begin to move. Energy in motion is emotion. Emotion that moves transforms. Emotion that is suppressed festers. Feel what you feel. All of it. That is where your healing lives.

Changing Your Energy

If everything is energy, and your thoughts and emotions are energy, then changing your life begins with changing your energy. This sounds simple but it is not always easy. However, it is always possible. The simplest way I know to change my energy is by dancing to my favorite music. The words in the song, the instruments, the voice of the singers. It doesn't have to be a happy, uplifting song. It can be dramatic and passionate. How does music make you feel? Do you notice if it changes your energy?

Here is what I know from years of clinical practice and personal healing: The most powerful way to shift your life is not to change your circumstances first; it is to change your internal state. When you change inside, the outside must follow. You have more power than you know. The question is whether you are willing to use it.

Energy Exercises

Exercise 1: The Energy Audit

For one week, keep a simple journal. At the end of each day, ask yourself: What raised my energy today? What drained it? What thoughts did I repeat most often? What emotions did I feel most frequently? At the end of the week, look for patterns. Your energy audit will show you exactly where your attention—and therefore your creative power—has been going.

Exercise 2: The Vibration Shift

When you notice your energy dropping—when fear, anxiety, or heaviness sets in—practice this: Stop. Place one hand on your heart. Take three deep breaths. Ask yourself, "What is the highest-frequency thought I can genuinely believe right now?" Find a real thought that feels true and feels better than where you are. Hold it. Feel it shift your body. Repeat as needed.

Exercise 3: Body Energy Scan

Lie down comfortably. Close your eyes. Starting at the top of your head, slowly scan your awareness down through your body. Where do you feel ease? Where do you feel tension, heaviness, or constriction? Don't try to fix anything. Just notice. Place your hand on any area that calls for attention. Breathe into it. Ask, "What are you holding? What do you need?" This practice, done consistently, will teach you to read your body's energy language.

Notes

I AM aware of my state.
I AM capable of shifting it.
I AM responsible for my response.

M: Meditation

The quieter you become, the more you are able to hear.

—Rumi

I want to tell you something that still surprises me when I say it out loud.

I am a doctor of chiropractic. I was pre-med at UC Davis, trained from the beginning to see the body through the lens of Western medicine. Diagnosis. Imaging. Prognosis. Structural reality. What science says. What the textbook says. What is and is not possible based on what shows up on a scan or x-ray. That was my first language. And for a long time, it was the only language in the room.

So when I broke my back at five months pregnant, that first language spoke immediately and clearly. I knew exactly what a broken back meant. I knew the anatomy. I knew the prognosis. I knew, better than most patients ever do, precisely what I was dealing with.

And in knowing all of that, I had already begun to build a ceiling around my own healing.

This is something nobody tells you about medical training. The knowledge that is meant to help you can also limit you—because when you know what something is supposed to mean, you can unconsciously organize your entire system around that meaning. Your beliefs become your biology. Your prognosis becomes your prison.

What cracked that ceiling open was not another medical intervention. It was meditation—specifically, visualization. Seeing my spine whole. Seeing my pelvis restructured and aligned. Seeing my body not as it was on the imaging but as I intended it to become.

I had been reading Dr. Joe Dispenza: his work on the mind-body connection, on how the brain cannot distinguish between a vividly imagined experience and a real one, on how sustained visualization literally begins to reorganize the body's chemistry and structure.[6] I had read it intellectually. And then I lived it. And everything changed.

Before the visualization breakthrough, the Zone Technique[7]—a healing method created by Dr. Peter Goldman, which I later became so passionate about that

---

6. Joe Dispenza, *Breaking the Habit of Being Yourself: How to Lose Your Mind and Create a New One* (Hay House, 2012).
Joe Dispenza, *You Are the Placebo: Making Your Mind Matter* (Hay House, 2014).

7. Mahsa Khodabakhsh, *Zone Technique: Your Path to Healing* (publisher, 2024).

I trained to master level and wrote the book on it for both doctors and patients[8]—had already begun doing something extraordinary. My pain was lifting in ways that defied what I thought I knew. I found myself moving more freely. Breathing more deeply. Two weeks of significantly reduced pain (with a broken back during pregnancy) when, by every Western medical measure, I should have been immobile and suffering.

Something in my thinking about my back was getting better. The Zone Technique was healing not just the injury but also the concepts I was holding around the injury. The fear. The ceiling. The quiet medical voice that kept reminding me what a broken back means. And then the visualization took over where the Zone Technique had begun. I would lie in stillness, close my eyes, and see—clearly, deliberately, with every ounce of focused intention I had—my spine perfect. My body whole. My back healed. My mind had been trained to see damage. I was reprogramming it to see possibility.

The proof came not in an X-ray or a clinical assessment. It came the day I found myself doing Ki aikido. Rolling on my back. Performing martial arts movements that if you had asked me months earlier, I would have told you were completely impossible for someone with my type of injury.

---

8. The Zone Technique was developed by Dr. Peter Goldman, based on the Zone Therapy principles of Dr. Thurman Fleet (1931). Dr. Mahsa Khodabakhsh is a Mastermind level practitioner and author of *Zone Technique: Your Path to Healing*.

The mind is not separate from the healing. It is the missing link. This chapter is about that link. About the practice that made it available to me. And about what becomes possible when you get quiet enough to let your body remember what it already knows how to do.

My First Real Meditation

I didn't know what to expect. I was nervous, genuinely nervous, in the way you are when you've agreed to something you can't quite picture.

It was Sara who invited me. She was my massage therapist, and her work had been part of my healing during a time when I needed it most. I had recently walked away from a career that looked extraordinary on paper—a position at LoopNet, financial security, a private company on the edge of going public—and I had walked away at twenty-six years old because something in me had been ignited that I could no longer ignore. I had chosen to go back to school. To study chiropractic. To follow the pull that made no practical sense and felt truer than anything else I had ever done.

One day on my way to my chiropractic adjustment appointment, my chiropractor, who had become a mentor to me, called me. "Mahsa, I want you to quit your job and come work for me" and so I had. This choice was completely led by intuition. Months had passed and I had left my corporate career and was now working in his office while I completed my prerequisite chemistry and physics classes for chiropractic school. Sara was the massage therapist who worked in this chiropractic office. We had great conversations, and she was ever so gentle with her technique, knowing that what I needed was more than just physical healing. Her life partner, Ananda, had spent nearly thirty years living and studying in an ashram, practicing and teaching a style of Tantric yoga and meditation I had never heard of. One evening, when Sara invited me to one of Ananda's meditation classes, I couldn't say no.

Before I walked into class that evening, Sara gave me a brief tutorial on the tantric breathwork technique. Inhale. Hold for a count of four. Swallow without exhaling. Inhale again immediately for another count of four. Then exhale, all the while imagining the breath moving up through the body, touching each energy center along the way. This was my first real introduction to the chakras. Ten minutes later, I was sitting on a meditation pillow in a quiet room with about twenty other students, certain I was going to do something wrong and embarrass myself in front of everybody.

The room settled. And then Ananda walked in.

He took his place on a small, raised platform—unhurried, completely still—and gently welcomed us. Then he opened his eyes. Slowly, deliberately, he looked at each student, barely moving his head, his gaze traveling around the room until it found mine. And when it found mine, I felt it. Not a look. A transmission. His eyes seemed to see me completely, and the energy behind them was unmistakable. Real. Alive. Unlike anything I had encountered before.

For twenty minutes, we breathed with our eyes open, holding his gaze, being held by it. Then we closed our eyes.

I was so focused on the breathing, running an inner dialogue with myself (*Am I doing this right? Am I holding too long? Is this correct?*), but then I felt it. A gentle but firm touch. One hand on the crown of my head. Another on my chest.

Boom.

A flow of light moved through my body. And with it came a message—not in words exactly, but in the way knowing arrives when it bypasses the mind entirely:

Your heart is broken. Heal your heart.

Tears began to fall softly down my cheeks. My throat tightened. Something in me wanted to cry out loud, a sound that had been waiting much longer than that evening to be released. I held it in and kept breathing.

After class, I walked up to Ananda. He recognized me from my doctor's office and smiled with a warmth that felt completely natural, completely unhurried.

"So nice to see you here. How did you like it?"

"It was amazing," I said shyly. "Very powerful."

"Come back next week. And if you can, come twice a week. It will be good for you."

I dropped a donation in the box by the door and walked out into the night. I didn't have a name for what had just happened. I only knew that something in me had been seen, something I hadn't even fully admitted to myself yet. And that whatever this practice was, it had reached a place that nothing else had reached.

The spirit within doesn't always wait for perfect conditions. Sometimes it simply waits for an open door. And that night, for the first time in a long time, mine had opened.

My Meditation Journey

I was not always someone who meditated.

For years, I was someone who did. Constantly. My identity was wrapped up in the doing: dancing, choreographing, performing, teaching, working, studying. Always moving. Always producing. Always becoming the next version of myself before I had finished meeting the current one. I wore my busyness like armor. If I stopped, I might have to feel what I had been running from.

And there was plenty to outrun. Michael's death. The grief I had never fully processed. The life I was trying to build on top of a foundation that hadn't yet healed.

After that first class with Ananda, I kept going back for years until I moved out of the area. Then I found Bikram yoga. Then Vinyasa. Then Iyengar. I loved everything about yoga, especially the end, laying in shavasana, when I felt my body vibrate and float the way it did when I danced.

I discovered the Esalen Institute[9] in Big Sur and began frequently attending their yoga and meditation retreats. During my four years earning my doctorate in chiropractic, I went one to two times per year. Those retreats were crucial support during some very challenging times in my life. Hidden blessings falling into my path for healing.

In my metaphysical minister's program, Dr. Paul Leon Masters, the founder and director of The University of Metaphysics, taught that a daily practice of meditation opens the surface levels of the mind to the deeper levels, where a higher consciousness exists that knows more about life as a whole than the intellect by itself could ever begin to fathom.[10] He dedicated over forty years to researching higher consciousness and discovered that when a person takes even a few minutes daily to meditate, the doorway of the mind remains open to an influx of what he called "extrasensory awareness." Through meditation, we stop relying solely on our intellect to guide our way and instead connect with a part of ourselves that holds the reason and purpose for which our soul incarnated into this lifetime.

---

9. Center for humanistic education and retreat, founded 1962.

10. Paul Leon Masters, *Spiritual Mind Power* (University of Metaphysics, 1978).

The Spirit Within

When you sit with yourself in stillness—alone or with others, eyes closed, breath steady, attention turned inward—something begins to happen. You remember the Spirit within you. Your inspiration. Your breath of life.

And this is what I believe our modern world has lost touch with: the Divine presence already living inside us. We look everywhere outside ourselves for healing, for direction, for peace, when so much of what we are seeking can be found in stillness.

Meditation taught me how to come home to myself. It taught me that I don't need to run from what I feel. I need to be present with it. And it taught me that the answers I was trying to find in books, classes, teachers, and relationships were already living inside me—I just needed to get quiet enough to hear them.

The Miracle of Your Body

The word *meditation* comes from the Latin *meditatum*, meaning "to ponder." So let's ponder, for a moment, about the body you live in.

Your heart is always beating without your command. Your lungs are exchanging oxygen and carbon dioxide without you remembering to make it happen. Your liver is detoxifying. Your kidneys are filtering. Your immune system is scanning, protecting, and repairing. All day. All night. Every day. For your entire life.

Your breath is not just air. It is life moving through you: Ki, chi, prana, Spirit made tangible. When you breathe consciously, you shift your physiology. You signal safety to your nervous system. You begin returning to regulation. What if, each day, you took one minute to feel gratitude for the body that carries your soul? Because gratitude changes you. Your internal state influences your chemistry, your nervous system, your immune response, and your capacity to heal.

The Spine Holds the Key

Your nervous system is an electrical communication network, sending and receiving signals between the brain and every cell, organ, and system in your body.

Let me give you a brief chiropractic history lesson. The founder of chiropractic, D. D. Palmer, was a healer and researcher. He was first a magnetic healer before he developed the chiropractic adjustment. He understood energy. He worked with life force. Through his research and practice, he came to understand the profound importance of the nervous system housed in the spine as the primary pathway through which our electrical energy, or our life force flows.

And yet, in just over a hundred years, thousands of years of wisdom that truly worked has been largely forgotten.

An entire civilization relinquished its trust in nature and handed it over to the laboratory.

The thread that has always resonated most deeply with me is this: There is an intelligence within you. It heals cuts. It coordinates digestion. It regulates hormones. It runs cellular repair. You do not have to consciously direct it, yet it is always working on your behalf. Meditation supports this system by reducing stress load, increasing body awareness, and helping you return to balance.

The I AM Presence

In the story where Moses encountered the Divine and asked for a name, the answer was: "I AM that I AM" (Exodus 3:14 NIV). Every time you say, "I AM," you invoke this same creative power. You are declaring the nature of your reality: *I AM worthy. I AM healed. I AM love. I AM enough.* These are invocations, calling forth the truth of your divine nature.

In meditation, you learn to rest in the I AM—the pure awareness before the labels, the stories, the identities. This awareness is your true self. It has never been wounded. It has never been broken. It is the part of you that is eternal, whole, loved and always at peace. The more time you spend here, the more that peace becomes the ground from which you live. And it begins with one practice: the sacred, daily act of getting quiet enough to hear yourself.

Meditation Exercises

Exercise 1: The Two-Minute Practice

If you have never meditated before, start here. Set a timer for two minutes. Sit comfortably. Close your eyes. Focus on your breath. When thoughts arise—and they will—simply notice them without following them, and gently return your attention to your breath. Two minutes. Every day. This is how transformation begins.

Exercise 2: The I AM Meditation (Ten Minutes)

Sit quietly and close your eyes. Take several deep breaths. As you settle, begin to repeat silently: *I AM.* Just those two words. With each inhale, *I.* With each exhale, *AM.* Feel the truth of your existence—not your story, not your roles, just the pure fact of your being. Rest here for ten minutes.

Exercise 3: The Morning Alignment (Five Minutes)

Before you check your phone, before you speak to anyone, before the day begins, take five minutes for yourself. Close your eyes. Take three deep breaths. Ask yourself: *Who am I choosing to be today? How do I want to feel? What is one intention I am setting for this day?* Sit with the answers. Let them settle into your body. Begin your day from this place.

Notes

P: Presence

When you walk into the presence of people who calibrate at the very highest energy levels, just being in their energy field, everything that is diseased or in disharmony is healed.

—Wayne Dyer

There is a particular quality of light that only exists right now. Not yesterday's light. Not tomorrow's. This light, falling at this angle, in this moment.

Your child is laughing in the next room. Your mother or father's voice on the phone. Your partner whispering in your ear, "I love you". The weight of a book in your hands. These moments don't announce themselves as precious. They simply pass, quietly and unremarkably, into memory. And one day, you will reach for them and find only the ghost of what was.

I say this not to create fear but to create wonder. Because when you truly feel how fleeting each moment is, presence stops being a discipline and becomes a gift you give yourself.

We are living in the first era of human history where presence has become an act of resistance. Our attention is under siege. Every notification, every ping, every scroll is designed to pull you out of the now and into a manufactured elsewhere. Technology companies employ neuroscientists and behavioral psychologists to engineer addiction to distraction! Your presence is being sold to the highest bidder—and most people don't even realize they're losing something irreplaceable.

Presence in My Practice

In my practice, being present with my patients was one of the most important skills I ever cultivated, and one of the most sacred responsibilities I carried.

There is so much being communicated that has nothing to do with words. Eye contact. The subtle tension in someone's shoulders. The way a person's voice changes when they finally say the thing they've been afraid to say. The energy they carry, and the way they walk into the room before they've spoken a single word. All of it tells you exactly what someone needs, if you are paying attention. And I learned early on that paying attention was not enough. I had to be fully there. I had to park everything outside that door and walk in with my listening ears, my seeing eyes, and my open heart.

Because when someone is truly present with you, you feel it. Your nervous system feels it: Your body relaxes. Your guard comes down. You feel safe enough to tell the truth about your pain, about your fears, about the things you haven't told anyone else. And that is when real healing can begin.

Time and time again in their testimonials, my patients wrote about one thing above all others: They knew they had my full attention. They felt loved. They felt cared for. So many of them told me they had felt dismissed in other settings, or rushed, like they were just a number. They came to me carrying not just their physical pain but also the pain of not being seen or heard. And I made it my mission to change that for every single person who walked through my doors.

I remember my dear patient David. He and his wife had recently moved to the area, and his previous chiropractor had referred him to me. I came to learn that David lived with a long-term liver condition and that his doctors had told him a transplant would eventually become necessary. For the first two years I saw him, he was doing beautifully. He was healthy. He was working on himself in every aspect: building his fitness, honing his strength, growing a beautiful family. And then, almost without warning, an unforeseen infection changed everything. His body began to shut down. He was suddenly in dire need of a donor.

You might wonder why a man with severe liver disease was sitting in a chiropractor's office. But for David, I was never really there to offer a modality. I was there to be a loving, supportive presence in his life. To hold his hand. To listen. To believe, with my whole heart, that he would heal, whether through the transplant he was waiting for or through some other grace neither of us could yet see. I was there to be a witness to his life.

By the grace of God, and some amazing surgeons and a wonderful loving donor, David survived. He received a healthy liver and began to thrive. And when he came back to see me, he said: "Your support and friendship was a huge part of my healing. I couldn't have made it without you." His survival and healing meant everything to me. It was one of the happiest memories of my life, probably right up there next to seeing my babies for the first time.

It was never about what I was trained to do. It was about being love for him. And presence, it turns out, is medicine.

Over the years in my practice, I lost patients to accidents, disease, death, and suicide. Each of those losses deepened something in me, a knowing that the time we have together is not guaranteed. That the presence we offer, the moment when someone finally feels truly seen and heard, matters in ways we cannot measure and may never fully know.

Presence is not a technique. It cannot be faked. It is love made tangible.

Being Versus Doing: The Observer Within

Eckhart Tolle wrote that most people live trapped in time—replaying the past or rehearsing the future, never fully inhabiting the only moment that actually exists: Now.[11] When I first read those words, something clicked. I realized I had been so caught up in *doing*—treating patients, running a business, raising children, managing a household—that I had forgotten how to simply *be*. And it took a while till I remembered.

Being is not passive. It is the most alive state there is. It is the awareness beneath all the activity, the consciousness that watches, notices, and feels. When you are in a state of being, you are fully *here*. Creation happens in the now. Healing happens in the now. Transformation happens in the now.

I had to learn this the hard way, through the people who needed me the most.

Presence with My Children

Earning the trust of my stepchildren was one of the most important things I have ever done. And I did not earn it through grand gestures or elaborate plans. I earned it through the simple act of presence: showing up for them, from the very beginning, so they could see that I would be a loving addition to their lives. When I met my step-kids,

11. Eckhart Tolle, *The Power of Now* (New World Library, 1997).

my stepson B. was twelve and my stepdaughter M. was nine years old. I knew and could see that similar to myself, they had suffered through their parents' separation and divorce. Being those delicate ages was hard enough, and now there was a new adult in their life. So I decided to show them my intentions by being a loving presence that they could count on.

To this day, my stepchildren and I have long, deep conversations because they know they can always come to me with anything and together we will find a solution. They know they will have my full attention. They know I will listen, I will be their witness, and that they are loved and accepted. Today B. is twenty-seven and engaged! And M. is twenty-four and graduated from university. I am so proud of both of them and my husband, and our beautiful blended family. And I will always have fond memories of our hang out sessions, late nights doing homework assignments, crying on my shoulder after break-ups or fights with their friends, or simply a late night talking about life. Our strong bond was built one present moment at a time.

My husband and I have two children together, D. and K. who are now in second and fourth grade, and they want nothing more than time with their Mama. To dance together. To play together. Or to sit side by side and read or simply be. When I put down my phone, when I stop thinking about work, when I turn toward them completely—I watch them light up. Because children always know the difference between a parent who is physically in the room and a parent who is truly with them. My children don't need me to be perfect. They need me to be present and a witness in their lives.

The Gift of Time

As our parents age, they want nothing more than our time: to sit with them, to listen to stories they've told a hundred times as though we are hearing them for the first, to be unhurried, to simply be there.

Because the window of being able to sit with the people who raised us, who still remember things about us that no one else will ever know, eventually closes. Sometimes quickly. Sometimes slowly. But it closes.

Presence is a practice of remembering what matters. The people in front of you. The moment you are in. The love that is available right now, if only you will stop and receive it.

Presence Is the Greatest Gift You Can Give

Think about what you want most from the people you love. To be seen. To be heard. To be felt. And when you give that, truly give it, something profound happens. You receive it too. Because when you are fully present with another person, you are also fully present with yourself. You are here. Alive. Connected. This is what it means to truly live.

Presence Exercises

Exercise 1: The Gap Practice

Set a timer to chime every hour throughout your day. When it sounds, stop whatever you're doing. Take three conscious breaths. Ask yourself: *Am I here right now, or am I lost in thought about the past or future?* If you notice you were lost in thought, simply come back. Feel your feet on the ground. Notice what you can see, hear, and touch. This trains you to catch yourself when you leave the now.

Exercise 2: The Observer Practice

For ten minutes each day, sit quietly and practice being the observer. Watch your thoughts like clouds passing through the sky. Don't engage with them, don't judge them, don't follow them. Just notice: *There's a thought about work. There's a worry about money. There's a memory from yesterday.* Practice the awareness that you are not the thoughts; you are the one watching the thoughts. This is where your freedom lives.

Exercise 3: The Presence Pledge

Choose one person in your life: a child, a parent, a partner, a friend. For one full week, every time you are with them, put your phone facedown and out of reach. Make eye contact. Listen without planning your response. Let them finish their sentences. Notice what shifts, in them and in you. Presence is a practice. And like all practices, it gets easier the more you do it.

Notes

O: Oneness

You and I are all as much continuous with the physical universe as a wave is continuous with the ocean.

—Alan Watts

It was spring in Iran, and also Persian New Year.[12] A month before my second birthday. My mother was pregnant with my sister.

We were at my great-grandmother's home celebrating Nowruz, and I was doing what toddlers do: running back and forth between play, my mother trying to feed me bites of food.

In between one of those bites, I ran outside to the backyard to see the goldfish in my great-grandmother's pond. Because it was cold, the pond was covered with a large tarp, and pinned down for winter.

12. This is called Norouz. It is the ancient Zoroastrian celebration of the spring equinox and Persian New Year.

I walked over and found an opening. Reaching for the goldfish with my tiny little hands, somehow, I lost my balance. Splash!

I fell into the pond. Under the tarp.

No one saw me. No one heard me.

My mom's uncle, Mr. Javadi, was using the outdoor restroom. When he walked past the pond, something stopped him.

He later told my mother: "I don't know why, but I felt as if I heard a voice; some inner knowing stopped me. I looked to the pond and heard the faintest splash. I walked over, saw a little opening, stuck my hand in, and pulled Mahsa out by her ankle."

I was drowning next to the beautiful red goldfish.

I believe that angels and guides—and the universal power that connects us all—used Mr. Javadi to save my life. The next day, from all the stress and worry of almost losing me, my mother went into labor and my baby sister was born: our little New Year's gift.

The Truth Beneath All Names

Throughout human history, across every continent, every culture has arrived at the same core understanding: There is one infinite intelligence that flows through all things. Some call it Source. Some call it the Universe. Some call it God. Some call it Consciousness. Some call it the Great Mystery.

The name doesn't matter. What matters is the truth beneath all the names: We are all expressions of this One.

Here is what took me years to understand: You cannot actually lose your connection to Source. A wave does not disconnect from the ocean when it rises; it simply forgets, for a moment, that it is water. You have never been disconnected. You have only, sometimes, forgotten what you are. And forgetting is human. Remembering is the practice.

I AM a Healer: The One Energy

From a young age, I learned to recognize this energy—this universal force that saved my life by the pond—and I learned that it flowed through me too.

I work with my hands. Healing for me comes through touch.

I remember being a small child, not more than three or four years old, sitting next to my Baba Bozorg Hossein—Grandpa Hossein—on a beautiful Persian rug laid outside on our patio in Iran. He had a lot of pain from various injuries, and although I was small, I knew that when I would sit next to him, hug him, kiss him, or just hold his hand, he would feel better.

My father was very athletic and played soccer. He would come home completely exhausted and in deep physical pain. Because I was young and smaller, he would ask me to walk on his back and massage his shoulders. Very quickly, I learned this alleviated his pain.

I slowly became more and more aware that through touch, through the use of my hands, I could help take away pain. But it wasn't just my hands. It was something flowing through my hands. Something bigger than me. Something I was connected to. The same force that moved through Mr. Javadi to save my life at the pond was now moving through me to help others heal. It is all *one* energy.

What Oneness Really Means

Oneness does not mean we are identical. It means we are interconnected.

Your healing ripples. Your regulation ripples. Your love ripples. When you calm your nervous system, you affect your children. When you choose presence, you affect your partner. When you heal your wounds, you alter the relational patterns of everyone around you.

We are participants in a shared human field. And every act of healing—however private, however quiet—ripples outward in ways we will never fully see.

Oneness Exercises

Exercise 1: The Interconnection Practice

For one week, practice seeing yourself in everyone and everything. When you look at another person, silently acknowledge: *You are me, in a different form.* When you see a tree: *You are me, expressing as a tree.* When you feel the sun: *You are me, expressing as warmth.* Notice how this practice shifts your experience. Notice how judgment softens. Notice how compassion arises naturally. Write about your discoveries.

Exercise 2: The Abundance Awareness Walk

Take a twenty-minute walk in nature, or even your neighborhood. Your only job is to notice abundance. Count how many leaves are on one tree. Notice how many blades of grass. How many birds are singing. How many colors are in the sky. How lavishly creation expresses itself. Feel this abundance. Let your body remember: *I am part of this. I am made of the same creative force that makes billions of flowers bloom every spring. Abundance is my natural state.*

Exercise 3: Source Connection Meditation (Ten Minutes)

Sit comfortably. Close your eyes. Place one hand on your heart. Take deep breaths. With each inhale, imagine you are breathing in light, energy, and life force from the Infinite Source. With each exhale, imagine any sense of separation dissolving. Repeat silently: *I am not separate. I am the Universe expressing itself. I am connected to all that is. I am held. I am loved. I am home.* Stay in this feeling for as long as you can.

Notes

W: Wisdom

Believe nothing, no matter where you read it, or who said it, no matter if I have said it, unless it agrees with your own reason and your own common sense.

—Buddha

Wisdom Is Remembered, Not Acquired

Society has confused wisdom with information. Schools give you degrees and call you educated. They fill your mind with supposed facts and call you intelligent. They hand you credentials and call you qualified. But I believe wisdom is something else entirely.

You were born with innate wisdom. It has been with you since the moment you took your first breath. It speaks to you constantly, in soft whispers, gentle nudges, quiet knowing. That feeling in your gut. That voice in your heart. That clarity that arises when you get still enough to listen. Your soul knows. Your body knows. The universal intelligence that created you flows through you every moment, guiding you, protecting you, showing you the way. But somewhere along the way, you learned to ignore it.

The Danger of Outsourcing Your Wisdom

Think about the first things you were taught to believe. Not facts you discovered yourself. Not truths you tested against your own experience. But things handed to you—by parents, teachers, religious leaders, culture—before you were old enough to question them. Most of us never go back and examine those beliefs. We simply carry them. Build our lives on them. Defend them as if they were ours, when really, they were given to us before we had the tools to choose.

Faith, at its purest, is not the absence of questions. It is the willingness to walk forward anyway, into the mystery, into the unknown, trusting that something greater is holding the path. That is very different from swallowing what your own soul knows to be wrong because someone with authority has told you to. One draws you closer to yourself. The other asks you to abandon yourself. You will always know the difference. Your body will tell you.

Fear: The Enemy of Wisdom

Fear is the greatest thief of wisdom. It whispers that you can't trust yourself. That your body is broken. That you need someone else to fix you. That without external intervention, you're doomed.

I learned this at nineteen years old.

I went to a doctor because my periods were irregular, a completely normal part of being a young woman, hormones fluctuating, my body still finding its rhythm. But the doctor looked at me with great concern and said: "If you don't take birth control to regulate your periods, you will never be able to have children."

Never be able to have children.

I was nineteen. I trusted the white coat. I believed that my body, which had been functioning perfectly well on its own for nineteen years, was broken and needed pharmaceutical intervention, or I would be infertile for life. So I took the pills. Out of fear. Because I didn't have access to my own wisdom yet.

I took those birth control pills for nine years. And they made me sick.

When I later studied human anatomy, physiology, nutrition, and toxicology in my doctoral program, I learned the truth. My body wasn't broken; it was communicating. I stopped the pills. I healed myself. I restored my body's natural intelligence. And when I later met doctors who truly understood fertility, they told me what my deeper knowing had always suspected: I was fully fertile. I always had been.

I gave birth to healthy, beautiful children. The doctor who scared me at nineteen was wrong. But I didn't know that then. I gave away my power because fear was louder than wisdom. And now I help others reclaim theirs.

When My Body Knew Before My Mind Did

There is a story I have never fully told. I share it now because it is the most visceral, undeniable proof I have of what wisdom—true, innate wisdom—actually feels like in the body.

It was three months after Michael died. I was twenty years old, working at a small restaurant in Rockridge, California, with my best friend, Mar—and it was exactly what I needed: distraction, movement, purpose, laughter. I was journaling constantly during this time. Writing to Michael. Writing to God. Asking the Universe why someone so full of light could be taken not just from me but from his family and our world. Using words on paper to pull the grief out of my body the only way I knew how.

Micheal's death wasn't just grief and loss for someone I loved, it was losing the one person who had made me truly feel I deserved to be loved, that I had nothing to be ashamed of, not where I was from, not my body, not for being a woman. Michael was a spiritual gift that taught me unconditional love, and in the short time of knowing him, he had healed wounds I was still too young to be able to identify or put into words. When he died, a large piece of my soul died with him. I started to doubt everything he loved about me. And days after his death, barely clinging to life myself, vulnerable and defeated, I became the perfect prey for a predator.

He was older, persuasive, controlling, and an alcoholic. I was young and naïve, and I did not yet know how to name what was happening to me, let alone how to escape it.

One evening, he paged me. When I called back, something in his voice stopped me. I can only describe it as a frequency: dark, tense, unpredictable. My body registered it immediately.

I sat in my car outside the restaurant and felt it—clearly, unmistakably—a knowing that I should not go back to his house that night. Not a thought. A physical sensation. As though the air itself was pressing against me, holding me in place. Every cell in my body speaking the same language: *Do not go.*

But my dog was there. My things were there. So I argued with my own wisdom. I overrode it. I drove there anyway.

The moment I pulled into the driveway, the feeling intensified into something I can only describe as arms—invisible, urgent—holding me back, whispering, *Don't go, don't go.* My heart was pounding the way an animal's does when it senses a predator. Everything in me knew.

And still I walked in.

The music was dark. Loud. Two empty wine bottles on the counter. I called his name into the silence. He was sitting in his live-work studio, reading my journal. He had a cigar in one hand, a glass of wine in the other. Pages marked. Pages torn.

What followed was one of the most violent nights of my life. He hit me with a book. He slammed my head into a cabinet. He forced wine down my throat. He beat me across my body with a broom handle. He sat on top of me, wrapped his hands around my throat, and told me he was going to kill me and burn the house down.

And in that moment—barely conscious, pinned to the floor, his hands around my neck—I looked directly into his eyes and said: "Good. Do it. So I can be with Michael."

He let go.

I don't know why. I only know that something in that surrender—that complete release of fear, that willingness to go—broke something in him. He stopped. I survived.

As I grew and healed, I came to understand what I could not see then: What happened was not my fault. I did not deserve it. He had no right to touch me. No right to go through my journals, the most private sanctuary I had, the place where I spoke to Michael, where I poured out my grief, where I was most vulnerable and most myself.

Abusive people are hurt people. Unhealed people. People who never learned to sit with their own pain. So they transfer it, weaponize it, direct it at whoever is closest. That does not excuse what he did.

What came next was a different kind of wound, one I was not prepared for.

I reached out. I asked for help, quietly, ashamed. I turned to women who were older than me, women who knew this men, women who had been there the very night my world collapsed, the night I learned Michael was gone. They had watched me break. They had seen me fold into a corner, sobbing, shattered. And they had walked past.

When I told them what happened, when I said the words out loud and asked what I should do, they had nothing for me. "Forget about it," they said. "Move on." One suggested, carefully, with a gentleness that still turns my stomach, that perhaps I had done something to bring it on, because he was an artist, he was passionate, so he lost it, big deal. One of them later pursued him.

I have sat with that for a long time. These were women at least eight to ten years older than me. Women who knew him, women who knew what I had just lost the night before he found me vulnerable and alone. And still, silence, deflection, blame.

The violence of this man's hands I could eventually understand. But the abandonment of women who knew? That took much longer to heal from. That cut differently.

I have asked myself what makes a woman turn away from another woman in her most broken moment. I believe it comes down to this: She has not yet faced her own pain. She has been taught by culture, religion, society, by every structure built to keep women small and separate, that another woman's suffering is inconvenient, or worse, a competition. That to validate her is somehow to diminish yourself.

But we were never meant to look away from each other. It is time to rise. To stand in the gap for one another. To say, clearly, and without hesitation, "This is not okay. You did not deserve this. I am not leaving you." This is not weakness, this is the most ancient form of strength we carry.

But I forgave him. It took years. The fear lived in my body long after the danger had passed, which is exactly what this chapter has been teaching you about trauma. It stores itself. It waits.

And here is what still makes me smile: my little dog Maloos carried the memory too, in her own way. She became extraordinarily sensitive to the smell of alcohol, to the energy of intoxicated people. She could detect it from a distance, and she would bark without stopping until they were gone. Sweet, fierce, loyal Maloos. She was my protector and my companion for sixteen years.

And at the end of her life, she chose my husband, Tim. She just adored him. He was gentle, kind, and patient with her. And somehow, that little dog who had been in that room that night, who had hidden and barked and trembled—she recognized in him something safe. Something good. Maloos knew. She always knew.

My body knew before I walked through that gate. My innate intelligence, that same force that heals cuts and regulates heartbeats and grows babies from nothing, was speaking to me in the only language it has: Sensation. Feeling. Knowing.

I didn't listen. Not because I was stupid or weak. I was twenty years old, drowning in grief, isolated, manipulated, and trapped in circumstances I didn't fully understand. That is what abuse does: It dismantles your access to your own wisdom slowly and methodically, until you can no longer trust what you feel.

Healing, for me, meant finding my way back to that knowing. Slowly. Painfully. Through years of work in my body, in meditation, in movement, in all the practices I have shared with you in this book. And now, when that feeling arises—that quiet, certain, cellular *no*—I listen. Every time. Without negotiation.

Your wisdom will never be louder than the moment you most need it. It will be a whisper. A weight in your chest. A tightening in your throat. A knowing that arrives before your mind has had time to think. That is the intelligence that has been protecting you your entire life.

Learn to hear it. Honor it. It may save your life.

Even Alternative Healing Can Use Fear

Fear-based manipulation doesn't only live in conventional medicine. This is something important and often overlooked.

When I became a chiropractor, there were messages in the field suggesting that people who weren't getting regular adjustments were suffering, degenerating, living below their full health potential. That they needed us, or they would never be truly well. I do not teach or practice from that place.

I have seen people whose bodies looked compromised on imaging, yet their souls were thriving, their nervous systems regulated, their spirits at peace. I met Tibetan war veterans with bullets still lodged in their spines who could sit in meditation for hours. I met a monk who slept on a hard marble floor so that the orphaned children he cared for could have comfortable beds. His spine, by chiropractic standards, should have been suffering. But he radiated joy. He moved with grace. He was whole in every way that mattered.

An x-ray can show bones, but it cannot show peace. An MRI can show tissue, but it cannot show purpose. True health is alignment: body, mind, and soul moving in harmony. Fear keeps you dependent. Wisdom sets you free.

Body Wisdom: Your Innate Intelligence

Your body is the wisest teacher you will ever have. It holds memories your conscious mind has forgotten. It speaks a language older than words: the language of sensation, instinct, knowing.

Long before your mind can rationalize or justify, your body tells the truth. The tightening in your chest when someone lies. The expansion in your heart when you are in alignment. The sinking feeling in your gut when something is wrong. This is wisdom, not anxiety.

One of the most powerful moments I witness in my practice is when someone finally reconnects with their body's wisdom. When they realize: *My body isn't broken. It has been trying to communicate with me. And I have been silencing it.* Your body is not your enemy. It has never been your enemy. It is your most loyal ally, your wisest teacher, and your most devoted healer.

Learning from My Grandfather

He was four years old when his mother died. The youngest of four children, left with a father who gambled away their inheritance and their future. My Baba Bozorg Asghar did whatever he could to help: cooking, cleaning, learning. At twelve years old, during World War II, he lied about his age and said he was sixteen so he could get work. He drove large trucks to the Russian border, trading for rice and food to help feed his family.

He worked hard his entire life. He lived simply. He loved deeply. My Baba Bozorg Asghar believed in the healing power of nature. He believed medicine came from the earth. He didn't set foot in a hospital until he was ninety-five years old.

For every meal, he made a big salad: cucumbers, red onions, tomatoes, fresh dill, mint, olive oil, and lemon juice. As he prepared it, he would tell me what each ingredient did for the body. In winter, he would sit with a pile of pomegranates in front of him, patiently peeling them until his hands were stained red, filling bowls for all the grandchildren. He had the biggest laugh, deep and full of life. He ran miles well into his old age.

The first time I gave him a chiropractic adjustment was at a family reunion we had in Turkey. It was also the last time I would see him. When I finished, he looked at me and told me I had great hands. He told me how proud he was that I was his granddaughter.

My Baba Bozorg Asghar transformed his wounds into wisdom. That is what integration looks like.

The Foundation of Empowerment

Wisdom is what emerges when you have walked through fire and chosen to extract meaning from the flames.

Your pain has taught you things no classroom ever could. Every betrayal showed you the value of trust. Every loss revealed what truly matters. Every moment you survived when you thought you couldn't taught you about your own resilience. True wisdom is not intellectual knowledge. It is embodied truth. It lives in your cells, in your bones, in the fabric of your being.

"The wound is the place where the Light enters you."[13]

Your cracks are not flaws. They are how the light gets in—and how the light gets out. You are not broken. You are broken open. There is a difference.

Wisdom Exercises

Exercise 1: Body Wisdom Dialogue (Seven Days)

Sit quietly and place your hand on your heart. Take three deep breaths. Then ask your body: *What do you need me to know right now?* Wait. Listen. The answer may come as a word, a feeling, an image, a sensation, or a knowing. Don't force it. Trust what arises. Write it down. Do this daily for seven days. Your body has been waiting to be heard.

Exercise 2: Innate Intelligence Tracking (One Week)

For one week, notice moments when your body heals itself without your conscious effort: a cut that closes, a headache

13. Jalal al-Din Rumi, *The Essential Rumi*, trans. Coleman Barks (HarperOne, 1995).

that passes, energy that returns after rest, sleep that restored you. Each evening, write down at least three examples of your innate intelligence in action. Gratitude amplifies this power.

Exercise 3: The Wisdom Question (Ongoing)

When faced with a decision, before consulting anyone else, sit in stillness and ask yourself: *What does my wisdom say? Not my fear. Not my ego. What does my knowing say?* Practice trusting this inner guidance before seeking external opinions. Your innate wisdom has been waiting for you to listen.

Notes

E: Evolution

There is no coming to consciousness without pain.
—Carl Jung

The True Meaning of Evolution

I didn't know back then what I know now. I had beliefs about myself that were holding me back from being me. I didn't feel worthy. Didn't feel good enough.

This was not my culture. My culture encompasses love, poetry, dance, the ancient Persian tradition of beauty and expression. Thank God for my culture, because that is what reminded me of love and the truth of where I came from.

No, these limiting beliefs came from the world I was born into, not by my choosing, and not by my family's choosing.

To understand what I mean, you have to understand what Persian women had only a generation before me, because most of the world has forgotten, or never knew. My mother came of age in an Iran that the news has never shown you. Iranian women won the right to vote and to stand for public office in 1963. To put that in context for you, this was eight years before the women of Switzerland could vote in their own country. Persian women were doctors, judges, senators, professors. By 1978, twenty-two women sat in parliament. One-third of university students were female. Two million women were in the workforce. The marriage age for girls was eighteen. A husband could no longer divorce his wife with a sentence or take a second wife without the court's permission. My mother walked through doors her own mother had only dreamed of.

Then, almost overnight, those doors began to close.

To understand what was lost, you have to understand what Iran *was*. My homeland is one of the oldest continuous civilizations on earth, a country of mountains and deserts and seas, of nomads and poets and merchants, of cities older than most nations. Within its borders live Persians, Azerbaijani Turks, Kurds, Lurs, Arabs, Baluch, Turkmen, speaking Persian, Azeri, Kurdish, Luri, Balochi, Arabic, and dozens of dialects between them.

And spiritually? Iran is a tapestry. Long before Islam ever arrived, Zoroastrianism was the faith of these lands, the faith of my ancestors, the faith that gave the world its earliest visions of one God, of light and darkness, of the sacred dignity of the human soul. The Magi were Persian. The word *paradise* itself comes from old Persian. Jews have lived on Persian soil since the sixth century B.C. Christians for nearly two thousand years. Sufis, mystics, Bahá'ís, Yarsanis, Mandaeans, each tradition adding another thread to the cloth.

This is the country my soul belongs to. Not a country of one God enforced by one ruler, but a country of many lights, many languages, and many ways of reaching the divine.

The Islamic Republic could not abide by that. Men who appointed themselves the guardians of God, men who decided they alone could speak for the divine, declared their version of Islam the only legitimate path. Anything else became suspect. Anything else became dangerous. To disagree was to be silenced. To dissent was, too often, to die. The religious tolerance that had characterized Iran under the monarchy came to an end with the revolution. The Zoroastrian community, keepers of Iran's most ancient spiritual heritage, fell from around 300,000 in the 1970s to roughly 20,000 today. The Bahá'ís, followers of a faith born on Persian soil, became the most persecuted religious community in the country. Poets, professors, students, ethnic minorities, women who refused the veil, anyone whose existence challenged the regime's grip on power could be imprisoned, tortured, or executed.

What was taken was not just rights, not just freedom, it was the soul of a nation.

The Islamic Republic was not something my parents welcomed or wanted for their children. It was forced upon an entire nation, and those of us born into it had no say in the world we were handed. With a stroke of a pen, the law that had protected women was suspended. The legal age of marriage for a girl was reduced from eighteen to nine. Women lost the right to seek a divorce and the right to custody of their own children. Female judges were dismissed. Women were eased out of government offices and barred from certain fields of study. The veil, once a personal choice, became a state-enforced uniform. The fundamentalist laws that followed told women how to cover their bodies, how to move, what to say, what to feel.

I want you to feel the velocity of that loss, because I felt it in my body before I had words for it. Imagine being a small girl in a country where, within your own mother's lifetime, women had been senators, and where now, the law required you to hide yourself in public before you were old enough to read.

That environment seeped into my consciousness anyway. It taught me to make myself small. To hide my body. To silence my voice. To shrink.

My parents didn't teach me this. My culture didn't teach me this. The oppression around me left marks. And this chapter is about what it took to outgrow them.

And yet, something in my heart and soul wanted me to be free.

So at times I would do something bold that would shock even me. It was as if something would take over, my soul breaking through the cage of my conditioning, and I was performing a dance for my entire high school, or reciting a poem in front of a crowd of a thousand. Something bigger than my fear was moving through me.

There were times I would lose my courage and fall again. Evolution is not a straight line.

And honestly? I am still nervous sometimes. Even now. But I push myself. The difference between who I was and who I am now is not the absence of fear; it's the willingness to move forward anyway. This is evolution. Not becoming fearless. Becoming willing.

Evolution is not about becoming someone you're not. It is about shedding everything you're not so you can reveal who you've always been.

You are not becoming empowered. You are remembering that you always were.

Evolution is part of the human experience. We are always growing. Through our experiences, we gain knowledge. We make mistakes, but we can learn from them. When we don't learn from them, we repeat them. But even still, we grow.

Michael Beckwith, founder of Agape International Spiritual Center, teaches that there are four stages of spiritual evolution: (1) life happening to you, the victim stage; (2) life happening by you, the manifester stage; (3) life happening through you, the channel stage; and (4) life happening as you, oneness with Source. The journey of I AM EMPOWER is the journey through all four stages: from feeling powerless, to reclaiming your creative power, to becoming a vessel for divine expression, to finally remembering that you ARE the Divine expressing itself.

The Heavy Coat

The most significant evolution of my life didn't happen in a meditation. It didn't happen in a therapy session or a yoga class or a moment of divine revelation.

It happened on a warm sunny Mother's Day at the Santa Cruz Beach Boardwalk, when I turned a corner and came face to face with the man who had nearly killed me twenty-five years before.

But let me back up.

A few years ago, I began experiencing inexplicable claustrophobia on airplanes. Completely out of nowhere. It made no sense to me; I had flown countless times without issue. So I called a colleague who practiced Rapid Transformational Therapy (RTT), and we set up a series of five sessions to find the root.

The sessions were powerful. I felt better. But something still wasn't quite resolved, and I couldn't identify what was underneath it—until one session, when the past abuse surfaced.

There I was, under hypnosis, and he was there—not physically, but present in the way things are present when the subconscious finally decides it is time. And for the first time in my life, I allowed myself to be angry. Not at myself. At him.

You see, somewhere along the way I had done what so many survivors do without realizing it: I had forgiven him while quietly continuing to blame myself. I thought I had processed it. I thought I had moved through it. But I had never once allowed myself to feel the full, clean, justified anger of someone who had been wronged.

So there I was, speaking out loud everything I had never said. Every word I had swallowed. Every truth I had been too afraid or too ashamed to voice. I said it all. And then, in the way of hypnotherapy, I imagined him gone. Erased. Every trace of him cleared from the landscape of my mind.

After the session, my colleague gave me a recording: a personalized audio to reprogram the subconscious mind, filled with positive intentions and the vision of the life I wanted to live. She instructed me to listen every night for twenty-one days. Every night, I would press play and fall asleep within five minutes.

Three days later, it was Mother's Day. My husband Tim and our children and I were at the Santa Cruz Beach Boardwalk—the ocean sparkling in front of us, the sun warm on our skin, the kids pulling us toward the rides. It was one of those ordinary, perfect days that you don't know you'll remember forever until you're already in the middle of it.

We turned a corner.

And there he was.

I knew instantly. Even after twenty-five years. Even with sunglasses on. I felt him recognize me at the same moment I recognized him. He walked past with a woman beside him, and I was holding my children's hands, and in my head, I heard myself saying, *Oh my God oh my God oh my God*—until I realized I was saying it out loud.

"What? What's wrong, honey?" Tim said.

"That was him. The one who hurt me when I was young."

Tim looked in the direction he had gone. "Are you okay? Should I go beat him up?"

I laughed—genuinely laughed. "Ha! Very funny. That would be a first." I took a breath. "No. It's okay. He's gone. I'm just so shocked. After twenty-five years. Just like that."

And then we kept walking. Into the sunshine. The kids swinging from our hands.

A few days later on my next RTT call I remembered to tell my colleague what had happened.

"Oh my God, Mahsa. You're kidding me right now."

"I know," I said. "Twenty-five years and there he was, just—"

"Wait," she interrupted. "The heavy coat."

"What heavy coat?"

"The recording, Mahsa. You fall asleep five minutes in, every night, but ten minutes in, I talk about him. I describe him as a heavy coat you've been wearing for years. A coat so familiar you forgot you had it on. And I tell you that on a hot, beautiful day at the beach, you finally take it off. You drop it on the sand. And you walk away and never look back."

Silence.

"Oh my God," I whispered.

"You were at the beach, Mahsa. On a hot, sunny day. With your children. And you dropped him there and kept walking."

The power of the subconscious mind. The intelligence of the universe. The way healing moves through us even while we sleep—doing its quiet, faithful work without our conscious permission or understanding.

I had forgiven him years before. But forgiveness without anger is incomplete. It is a door left slightly ajar. That RTT session let me feel what I had never allowed myself to feel—

the clean, righteous anger of someone who deserved better and finally knew it. And then the universe, in its mysterious and precise way, delivered the moment of completion.

A warm day. A beach. My children's hands in mine. My husband beside me, making me laugh. The heavy coat, dropped on the sand.

This is what evolution looks like. A slow, faithful, sometimes surprising unwinding, until one day, you turn a corner and realize that what used to have power over you simply doesn't anymore. You kept walking. That's all. You just kept walking.

And that—that is everything.

Worthiness: Remembering What You Forgot

Have you ever felt that you were not worthy of love? Of abundance? Of the life you secretly desire?

Here is a truth that will change your life: you are not separate from the Creative Source. You *are* an expression of it. The same intelligence that creates galaxies, orchestrates seasons, and grows forests from seeds is the intelligence expressing itself as you. When you deny your worthiness, you deny the divinity within you.

Worthiness is not something you earn; it is something you remember. You were born worthy. Somewhere along the way, the world offered you a different story about yourself. And because you were young, and because the people telling it seemed certain, you believed them. But a story is not a truth. And you are allowed, at any point, to set it down.

Shedding Identity to Find Your True Self

Your true self has been buried under layers of identity. Labels, roles, beliefs, and stories that you've accumulated throughout your life. *I am a mother. I am a victim. I am successful. I am damaged.*

There is nothing wrong with these identities; they serve a purpose in navigating the physical world. But they are not who you *are*. When you identify completely with these roles and labels, you forget your true nature. Who are you without your name? Without your job title? Without your past? Without your wounds? Strip away every label, every role, every belief about yourself. What remains? That is your true self. That is the I AM presence. That is pure consciousness, temporarily housed in form.

The Shoes That No Longer Fit

As a child, when you grew out of a pair of shoes, you were never able to fit into them again. Think of your growth in other areas the same way.

Once you expand your consciousness, once you learn a truth, once you embody a new level of awareness, you cannot unknow it. You cannot shrink back into who you were before. Old patterns might call to you, but you will feel the constriction. Those old shoes no longer fit. Trust this discomfort. It is proof of your evolution.

What Evolved Consciousness Actually Feels Like

Since I was a child, I have always felt a very deep connection to a higher power. I always asked to be guided to my purpose, to find strength in dark times and to do the work my soul was sent here to do.

And here's the thing—I never felt it was for me alone. I wanted it for everyone. For the people in Iran. For those living in poverty across the world. For the orphaned children. For the animals without warmth, shelter, and food. For the trees being cut down without new ones planted. For the earth herself. My heart aches. It still aches.

I felt the energy in a rock in the middle of my path. I felt the pain of a branch on a tree. And I still do. This is what evolved consciousness feels like. It's not detachment. It's feeling everything. It's being so connected to the web of life that you can't separate your own well-being from the well-being of all beings.

Evolution is the expansion of love until there is nothing left outside of it.

Evolution Exercises

Exercise 1: The Identity Excavation

Take your journal and write, "I AM . . ." at the top of the page. Now list every identity you hold—parent, child, professional, victim, survivor, healer, and so on. Write them all. Now, one by one, cross each one out while saying aloud: "I am not [identity]. I am the one who experiences being [identity]." When you've crossed them all out, sit in the silence. Who are you without all these labels? Write down what you feel, sense, or know in this spaciousness. This is your true self beginning to emerge.

Exercise 2: Soul-Purpose Dialogue

In a meditative state, ask your soul: *What did you come here to learn? What did you come here to give?* Wait in the silence. The answer may come as words, images, feelings, or simply a knowing. Write down whatever arises without judgment. Do this practice monthly. As you evolve, your understanding of your soul's purpose will deepen and clarify.

Exercise 3: Future Self Meditation (Ten Minutes)

Sit comfortably and close your eyes. Take several deep breaths. Imagine yourself one year from now, having evolved into your highest version, not in terms of accomplishments, but in terms of consciousness. See how this version of you carries themselves, how they speak, how they respond to challenges. Feel the peace, the power, the presence. Now ask this evolved self: *What do I need to know? What do I need to release?* Listen. Write down what you receive. Do this weekly and watch your consciousness expand.

Notes

R: Reveal

I wish I could show you when you are lonely or in darkness the astonishing light of your own being.

—Hafiz of Shiraz

I AM willing to grow.
I AM responsible for my choices.
I AM not my fear.
I AM not my past.
I AM evolving into wholeness.
I AM EMPOWER.

You made it. Not to the end. To the beginning.

Everything you've learned through energy, meditation, presence, oneness, wisdom, and evolution has prepared you for this moment. The moment when you stop doing the inner work in private and start living it out loud.

This is where it gets real. This is where it gets uncomfortable. This is where most people turn back. Because *reveal* is not about understanding yourself better. It's about taking everything you've discovered about who you truly are—and letting the world see it.

The Dance: From Suppression to Expression to Liberation

I was a child when I first felt the pull to move my body. Dance was already alive in me, even then, moving through my limbs, begging for expression. But I learned quickly that my body wasn't mine to express freely.

In the Iran I grew up in, a woman's body was not her own. The laws imposed upon us—not by our culture, not by our people, but by a government that had seized control of everything, including how we moved—made expression dangerous. Showing your body could bring punishment. It could bring shame upon your family. In the worst moments of that era, it could cost you your life.

So I danced at home. Behind closed doors. In secret. Where no one could see.

My parents always knew we wouldn't stay. They were not willing to raise two daughters under that regime, under those fundamentalist laws. So they were willing to sacrifice everything: their family, their home, the only life they had ever known. They were willing to start again. My mother wanted to study. My father wanted his wife and his girls to live without restrictions, without fear, without asking anyone's permission. We had family in Washington, D.C., and in California. It would be one or the other.

I still remember going with my mother and my sister to the American embassy for our visa interview. I had been practicing my English nonstop for weeks, so determined to get it right. When it was my turn, the kind woman behind the glass smiled at me and said, "Hello." And I said, "Hello." She said, "How are you?" And I said, "How are you?" She said, "What's your name?" And I said, "What's your name?" Word for word, like a little parrot. She started laughing. And she gave us a visa.

We came first, my mother, my sister, and me. My father stayed behind to close the life we had been living. While we settled in, my parents began the process of filing for political asylum. A year later, my father joined us. Eventually, after a long road, we were granted residency. And later still came the day I will never forget, the day we became American citizens.

I tell you this because I want you to feel what it took to get here. The leaving. The waiting. The faith of two parents who chose, against everything familiar, to give their daughters a future where their bodies and their voices could be their own.

And now, finally, I could dance.

Publicly. Freely. Without fear. I came alive.

Dance wasn't something I learned; it was something I remembered. Something that had been waiting, dormant, hidden, for permission to finally emerge. I didn't just take classes. I became a teacher. A choreographer. A performer. I cofounded a nonprofit dedicated to sharing Iranian American culture through art and aesthetics.

I thought I was free. I thought the fear was behind me. But then the judgment came—not from a regime this time, but from my own community. Here's the irony that still takes my breath away: I escaped Iran to be free. And then, as a young adult pouring my heart into preserving the beauty of Persian dance and culture, I faced the exact same suppression—this time from people who claimed to be educated, upper class, liberated. They called my dancing inappropriate. Shameful. They said a good, proper woman didn't move like that.

I eventually walked away from the organization I had founded. I let them drive me out. I made myself small to accommodate their discomfort.

But let me tell you what I understand now that I didn't understand then: They were doing the best they could with what they knew. They were modeling what they had been taught, behaving from their own egos and insecurities, their own unhealed wounds. People who have forgotten their own light will always feel threatened by someone else's.

And because I was still learning to see my own worth, I made myself smaller. I accepted their crumbs. I gave away my power. But today? Today I will not hold anything back. Today I will be seen. I will be heard. I will not make myself small because other people are uncomfortable.

We were built to move our bodies. Our physical form was designed for expression, for rhythm, for connection, for power. Dance is a communal expression. We were meant to move together. To witness each other. To celebrate the body as the sacred vessel it is.

I AM *revealed.* And so are you.

The Prison of Hiding

For too long, you've kept your true self locked away. You learned early that it wasn't safe to be fully you.

Maybe your family needed you smaller, quieter, more compliant. Maybe your religion told you your natural expression was sinful. Maybe past relationships punished you for being too much—too sensitive, too intense, too powerful, too different, too ambitious, too wild. So you adapted. You performed. You created a version of yourself that was acceptable, digestible, safe. But your soul never forgot.

Think about the versions of yourself you have performed over the years. The one who never caused problems. The one who never asked for help. The one who made herself plain so that others would feel comfortable. The one who achieved endlessly to prove she deserved to exist. The one who gave everything and kept nothing. Each of these was born from a moment when you decided, consciously or not, that the real you was too much.

And it worked. For a while. But a soul cannot live indefinitely in a costume. Eventually, it begins to press against the seams. Eventually, it finds a way to breathe—through your art, your anger, your grief, your longing, your inexplicable sense that there must be more than this.

That pressing? That longing? That is your true self, reminding you that it is still there. Now is when you unlock the door. Now is when you step out of the shadows. Now is when you let your soul finally, fully, shine.

Why Reveal Matters: Your Soul's Assignment

When you hide yourself, you're not just playing small for comfort. You're blocking your destiny. You're preventing your purpose from unfolding. You're denying the world the medicine only you can bring.

The parts of yourself you've been most afraid to reveal? Those are exactly the parts the world is waiting for. That sensitivity you tried to toughen up—someone needs your empathy. That intensity you tried to tone down—someone needs your passion. That truth you've been afraid to speak—someone needs to hear it to set themselves free.

Your soul didn't come here to blend in. It came here to shine. To disrupt. To transform. To show others what's possible when you stop hiding and start revealing. The world doesn't need another version of who you think you should be. It needs you. The real you. The powerful, unapologetic you. And it starts the moment you decide: I will hide no more.

The Work of Revelation

Revealing yourself is not a onetime event. It's a practice. A daily choice. A sacred commitment. Speaking your truth even when your voice shakes. Setting boundaries without apology. Showing your emotions instead of performing strength. Claiming your power without dimming it. Living your values, even when they're unpopular. Being visible even when visibility feels vulnerable.

This is the hardest work you'll ever do. Because every time you reveal yourself, you risk rejection. Judgment. Loss. That fear is real. That risk is real.

But the cost of hiding is greater than the risk of revealing. When you hide, you lose yourself. When you reveal, you gain the only thing that truly matters: your life. Your real life. The one your soul came here to live.

Reveal Exercises

Exercise 1: The Mirror of Truth (Daily—Five Minutes)

Every morning, stand in front of a mirror. Look yourself directly in the eyes. Place both hands on your heart and declare: *I AM divine. I AM powerful. I AM worthy. I AM revealed.* Do this every morning for forty days. Your entire energy will shift.

Exercise 2: The Sacred No (Weekly)

Practice saying *no* to anything that diminishes your divine nature: no to relationships that don't honor you, no to work that doesn't value you, no to anyone who wants you small. Each no is an act of self-love. Each no makes space for your yes.

Exercise 3: The Visibility Vow (Monthly)

Once a month, do something that makes you visible in a way that previously scared you: Share your truth publicly, wear something that makes you feel powerful, express yourself unapologetically, claim your power in a space where you've been small. Document how it feels. Watch yourself become free.

Notes

I AM no longer hiding.
I AM no longer small.
I AM divine.
I AM powerful.
I AM worthy.
I will not apologize for my light.
I AM revealed.

Conclusion

You Are the One You've Been Waiting For

You made it. Not to the end of a book. To the beginning of your life. The life you were always meant to live. The life your soul has been waiting for. The life that becomes possible when you finally remember who you are.

The Journey You've Taken

You began with energy—discovering that you are not just flesh and bone, but a vibrational being made of the same force that moves the stars and grows the forests. You learned that your thoughts, words, and emotions are constantly creating your reality.

You moved into meditation—the sacred practice of getting quiet enough to hear your soul, to connect with the I AM presence that has always lived within you.

You explored presence—learning that the greatest gift you can give is your full attention, your open heart, your willingness to truly be with yourself and others in this moment.

You remembered oneness—the truth that we are not separate beings bumping into each other on a random planet, but one consciousness expressing itself through infinite forms. What you do to another, you do to yourself. What you heal in yourself, you heal in the world.

You reclaimed wisdom—the innate knowledge that lives in your bones, your gut, your heart. The wisdom you were born with. The wisdom that was never lost, only forgotten.

You embraced evolution—understanding that your soul came here to grow, to shed old identities, to become more of who you truly are. That your struggles were not punishments but preparation.

And finally, you chose to reveal—to step out of hiding, to take off the masks, to let the world see the divine being you have always been.

This is the journey of I AM EMPOWER. And now it lives in you.

The World I Pray For

I always asked to be guided to my purpose, to do the work my soul was sent here to do.

I feel your longing to be free. Your desire to be seen. Your readiness to step into your power. And I pray for a day when so many have evolved their consciousness and evolved in their ability to love. Can you imagine the world we would live in?

A world where each person recognized the I AM within themselves and within every other being. A world where we stopped harming each other because we understood that harming another is harming ourselves. One person at a time. One awakening at a time. One choice to love instead of fear at a time. You are part of this collective evolution.

The Truth You Now Carry

You are not broken. You never were. You are not unworthy. You never were. You are not powerless. You never were.

You are a divine being who temporarily forgot your divinity. And now you remember.

You are energy—pure creative force.

You are meditation—connected to infinite intelligence.

You are presence—fully alive in this moment.

You are oneness—inseparable from all that is.

You are wisdom—guided by your innate knowing.

You are evolution—always growing, always becoming.

You are revealed—no longer hiding, finally free.

You are EMPOWER.

A Blessing for Your Journey

As you close this book and step forward into your life, I offer you this blessing:

May you never again forget who you are. May you trust your body's wisdom and your soul's knowing. May you speak your truth, even when your voice shakes. May you set boundaries without apology and love without reservation. May you feel the energy that connects all things and know you are never alone. May you meditate not to escape your life, but to create it. May you be fully present—with yourself, with those you love, with this precious moment that will never come again. May you see the divine in every being you encounter, even those who have forgotten it in themselves. May you transform your wounds into wisdom and your pain into purpose. May you evolve beyond every limitation you've ever accepted and become more of who you truly are. May you reveal yourself fully—your light, your shadow, your power, your love—without apology, without shame, without fear.

And may you always remember:

I AM EMPOWER.

The Declaration

Stand up. Place your hands on your heart. And say these words out loud:

"I AM divine. I AM powerful. I AM worthy of love, respect, and adoration.

"I AM no longer hiding. I AM no longer small. I AM no longer giving my power away.

"I AM energy. I AM meditation. I AM presence. I AM oneness. I AM wisdom. I AM evolution. I AM revealed.

"I AM EMPOWER."

And so it is.

One Final Truth

You picked up this book because something in you was ready. Ready to heal. Ready to grow. Ready to remember. That something was your soul. Your soul led you here. Your soul knew you were ready. Your soul has been waiting for this moment.

You are the one you've been waiting for.

The power has always been within you. The wisdom has always been within you. The divine has always been within you. This book simply helped you remember what you already knew. Now go live it.

Love heals. And you are love!

Go be the energy you want to see in the world. Go embody the presence you wish others would give you. Go love with the fierceness of someone who knows they are love itself. Go shine so brightly that others remember they have permission to shine too.

The world needs you. The real you. The empowered you. The revealed you. Not someday.

NOW.

I AM EMPOWER.

And so are you.

Forever.

With all my love,
Dr. Mahsa

Recommended Reading

Beckwith, Michael Bernard. *Spiritual Liberation: Fulfilling Your Soul's Potential.* Agape Media International, 2008.

Dispenza, Joe. Breaking the Habit of Being Yourself: How to Lose Your Mind and Create a New One. Hay House, 2012.

Hay, Louise L. You Can Heal Your Life. Hay House, 1984.

Lipton, Bruce H. The Biology of Belief. Hay House, 2005.

Myss, Caroline. Anatomy of the Spirit. Harmony Books, 1996.

Northrup, Christiane. Women's Bodies, Women's Wisdom. Bantam Books, 1994.

Pert, Candace B. Molecules of Emotion. Scribner, 1997.

Rumi, Jalal al-Din. The Soul of Rumi: A New Collection of Ecstatic Poems. Translated by Coleman Barks. HarperOne, 2001.

Van der Kolk, Bessel. The Body Keeps the Score. Viking, 2014.

Williamson, Marianne. A Return to Love: Reflections on the Principles of A Course in Miracles. HarperCollins, 1992.

Every teacher named in these pages pointed toward the same truth: the power to heal, grow, and remember who you are has always lived within you. These works are doorways. You are the destination.

—Dr. Mahsa

Here's What To Do Next

Closing this book isn't the end of the work, it's just the beginning! When you're ready, here are four ways we can keep going together.

1. Get Your Free Guide Keep the momentum going with *From Hustle to Wholeness*, my free companion guide to help you slow down and be in the now along with a guided breathwork session. Take it one day at a time.

Visit [https://youtu.be/3R_1Z5ytqRw?si=EiwJQASuzMWRTVyz] to download it free and stay connected to everything I share.

2. Go Deeper With Me If you want a guided path forward to E.M.P.O.W.E.R., there are two ways to step in. The *I AM EMPOWER* 90-day group program is where we do this work together in a private community. And for those who desire to be held more closely, and truly step into their truth, my private mentorship LOVE Redefined ™ is a one-on-one journey through Heal, Embody, and Radiate.

Visit [www.drmahsa.com] to explore both and find your fit, or schedule a call with me directly.

3. Invite Me to Speak If you are gathering people who are ready to step into their own power, I would be honored to bring this message to your stage, retreat, or event.

Email [info@drmahsa.com] with "SPEAKING" in the subject line.

4. Let's Stay Connected The conversation doesn't end here. Come find me on Instagram at [@dr.mahsakhoda], where I share daily reflections, and bring your story with you.

Acknowledgments

Let me begin by expressing so much love and gratitude to all the beautiful beings who have been my cheerleaders through every creative endeavor — my coaches and mentors, who saw what was possible in me and helped me break through to it.

And if you are reading this book, I thank you, too. It is because of you that I wrote it — to spark in you the sacred flame you carry deep within your heart. May you heal your pain and live your life in passion, empowered!

To my wonderfully goofy husband, Tim, who is always either making me laugh or crying right alongside me — thank you for encouraging me to tell my stories. I love you. I couldn't have done it without you.

To my beautiful children, Bailey, McKenna, Delara, and Kayan — may you move through this world empowered, always remembering that everything you could ever need already lives within you. I love you crazy and always have your back.

To my dear parents — thank you for the sacrifices you made to give me a life and freedom. And if you read this book, please know that I am healed, I am empowered, and I am loved.

To my dog Maloos, my companion of sixteen years through every struggle, I couldn't have survived without you, and thank you for picking Tim! To my dogs, Chiro, Cleo, I miss you every day. To my Mini, Summer, Milo, and Coco Chanel — you make the world a better place. Thank you for being my dogs!

And finally, to Michael — it all started with your love. I am forever thankful.

About the author

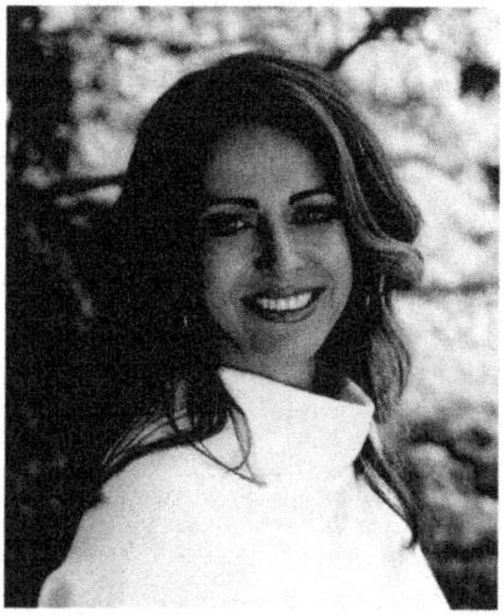

Dr. Mahsa Khodabakhsh is a Metaphysical Minister, Spiritual Teacher, author, and board-certified Doctor of Chiropractic. For nearly two decades, she has guided her patients and clients in healing and empowerment, teaching them to listen to their bodies, master their minds, and remember their spirit. Her work is a true integration of holistic medicine, somatic healing, and cognitive transformation, treating the whole human being as one inseparable miraculous system.

Born in Iran and raised in the United States, Dr. Mahsa came of age between two cultures. From the writings of Rumi, Hafez, and Paulo Coelho, to the ancient wisdom of the Persian magi and Zoroastrian mystics, and the modern science of mind-body healing, she grew up searching for the answer to one question: what truly heals a human being? Her search shaped an approach that bridges science, spirituality, and intuition combined with compassion, love, and empowerment to create lasting transformation. Her core message is the one she has lived: love heals, and you are love.

In her book I AM EMPOWER: The Path from Trauma to Truth, Dr. Mahsa shares the practical tools and personal stories that carried her through trauma, grief, and reclamation. Built around the EMPOWER framework — Energy, Meditation, Presence, Oneness, Wisdom, Evolution, Reveal — the book is a guide for anyone ready to move from the pain of their past into the freedom of their fullest self-expression. Dr. Mahsa lives in the San Francisco Bay Area with her family.

Made in the USA
Monee, IL
04 November 2026

67378029R00066